ROCK SOLID

A Guide to Being the Dad Your Kids Need

Robert A Reader

TABLE OF CONTENTS

INTRODUCTION

Rock Solid: A Guide to Being the Dad Your Kids Need by Robert A. Reader is more than just a book,it's a heartfelt journey into the depths of fatherhood and the fundamental principles that underscore effective parenting. With a blend of personal stories, expert insights, and timeless wisdom, Reader navigates the essential qualities and actions that define a supportive and reliable father figure.

This book serves as a comprehensive roadmap for fathers, offering guidance on how to strengthen their bond with their children and become the bedrock of their family's stability and growth. Whether it's tackling the challenges of discipline, fostering open communication, or nurturing emotional intelligence, Rock Solid provides the tools and perspectives necessary to cultivate a legacy of love, guidance, and resilience in the lives of your children.

Through practical advice and inspiring anecdotes, Rock Solid empowers fathers to embrace their role with confidence, compassion, and unwavering dedication. It's a guide that not only equips fathers with the skills they need but also inspires them to step into their role with authenticity and purpose, ensuring that they can truly be the dad their kids need.

CHAPTER 1: The Foundation of Fatherhood

In this chapter, we embark on a profound exploration of the foundational pillars of fatherhood, understanding that these principles serve as the bedrock upon which the relationships with our children are built.

Understanding Your Role

At the core of fatherhood lies a deep understanding of our role in our children's lives. It extends far beyond the provision of material necessities, it encompasses emotional support, guidance, and the unwavering embrace of unconditional love. By acknowledging the significance of our presence and influence, we lay the groundwork for shaping our children's development, nurturing their sense of security, and fostering a profound sense of belonging.

Setting Boundaries and Expectations

Central to effective parenting are clear boundaries and well defined expectations. These serve as essential guideposts, offering structure and predictability in our children's lives. By establishing rules with empathy and understanding, we create an environment of stability and consistency. Through the enforcement of boundaries, tempered with compassion, we not only instill discipline but also cultivate mutual respect and trust within the parent child relationship.

Being Present and Engaged

True presence transcends mere physical proximity; it entails a deep and sustained engagement with our children. In an era marked by relentless busyness, carving out dedicated time for meaningful interactions with our kids becomes paramount. Whether it's through the shared joy of bedtime stories, the laughter of playtime, or the earnest exchange of thoughts and emotions, being present allows us to forge bonds of genuine connection. In these moments, we affirm our children's worth, validating their experiences, and nurturing a profound sense of belonging.

Cultivating Empathy and Compassion

At the heart of every meaningful relationship lies empathy—the ability to understand and resonate with another's emotions. Cultivating empathy within our interactions with our children is fundamental to fostering healthy connections. By actively listening to their perspectives, validating their feelings, and responding with compassion, we impart invaluable lessons in empathy. Through our own actions and words, we model the transformative power of empathy, instilling in our children a profound appreciation for kindness, understanding, and the enduring bonds that unite us.

In essence, by embracing these foundational principles of fatherhood, we not only lay the groundwork for nurturing relationships with our children but also shape the course of their lives with wisdom, compassion, and unwavering love.

Prioritizing Self-Care

In the vast landscape of fatherhood, it's imperative to recognize that caring for oneself is not an act of selfishness but rather a fundamental necessity for overall well-being. As fathers, we are the pillars upon which our families lean, and to sustain that support, we must prioritize our own self-care. Whether it's dedicating time to physical exercise, indulging in hobbies that bring joy, or simply carving out moments of solitude to recharge, self-care is paramount for maintaining optimal physical, emotional, and mental health.

By prioritizing self-care, we not only replenish our own reserves but also set a powerful example for our children. Through our actions, we convey the importance of nurturing oneself in order to be fully present and engaged in the roles we undertake. In demonstrating the value of self-care, we impart a vital lesson—that investing in our own well-being ultimately enhances our capacity to be the best parents we can be.

Conclusion

In essence, the journey of fatherhood is a deeply enriching endeavor—one that is built upon a sturdy foundation of understanding, presence, empathy, and self-care. By embracing these core principles with intentionality and commitment, we pave the way for profound and enduring relationships with our children. So, let us nurture these essential elements with care and dedication, knowing that with each step, our foundation as fathers grows stronger, resilient, and evermore steadfast.

Nurturing Bonds with Your Kids

In the intricate tapestry of fatherhood, nurturing bonds with our children stands as a cornerstone—an endeavor that transcends mere presence to embrace the essence of connection, trust, and unwavering love. In this chapter, we embark on a journey to explore the profound significance of fostering these bonds and discover practical avenues to fortify the relationship between father and child.

Quality Time Matters

Within the bustling cadence of daily life, the gift of quality time holds immeasurable value. It's in these moments be it shared adventures, heartfelt conversations, or the simple joy of being together that the fabric of our bond with our children is woven. Make a conscious effort to carve out dedicated time amidst the clamor of responsibilities, prioritizing meaningful interactions that nourish the soul and deepen the connection between father and child.

Open Communication is Key

At the heart of every meaningful relationship lies the currency of communication an exchange that transcends words to encompass understanding, empathy, and trust. Foster an environment of open dialogue where your children feel empowered to express themselves freely, knowing that their voices are heard and valued. Cultivate the art of active listening, embracing their joys, fears, and aspirations with unwavering support and compassion.

Show Unconditional Love

In the grand tapestry of parenthood, unconditional love stands as the vibrant thread that binds hearts together in an unbreakable bond. Shower your children with expressions of love and affection, both in words and deeds, reaffirming that your love knows no bounds or conditions. Let them bask in the warmth of your embrace, knowing that in your eyes, they are cherished beyond measure, flaws and all.

Be Their Cheerleader

As fathers, we possess the unique privilege of standing as our children's staunchest allies and most fervent supporters. Celebrate their triumphs with unbridled enthusiasm, offering words of encouragement and applause as they navigate the winding path of life. In moments of adversity, be the beacon of hope and strength that guides them through the storm, instilling in them a resilient spirit and unwavering confidence in their abilities.

In essence, the art of nurturing bonds with our children transcends the realm of duty to embrace the essence of love, empathy, and understanding. Through quality time, open communication, unconditional love, and unwavering support, we lay the foundation for relationships that stand the test of time—forged in the crucible of shared experiences, mutual respect, and boundless affection.

Lead with Empathy and Understanding

In the intricate dance of fatherhood, empathy emerges as the guiding light—a beacon of understanding that illuminates the path to profound connection and mutual respect. In this section, we delve into the transformative power of empathy and its pivotal role in nurturing bonds with our children.

Empathy: The Bridge of Understanding

Empathy serves as the bridge that traverses the chasm between hearts, fostering a deep sense of connection and understanding. Step into your children's shoes, embracing their joys, fears, and struggles as if they were your own. Validate their emotions with sincerity and compassion, offering a safe harbor in which they can express themselves freely. By extending empathy in your interactions, you cultivate an environment of trust and acceptance, laying the groundwork for a resilient and enduring bond.

Patience in Practice

In the ebb and flow of parenthood, patience emerges as a steadfast companion—a virtue that softens the edges of frustration and tempers the trials of disagreement. Show understanding and forbearance, even in moments of tension or discord. Approach challenges with a calm demeanor, seeking to understand before seeking to be understood. By exemplifying patience, you not only strengthen the emotional fabric of your relationship but also impart invaluable lessons in grace and resilience.

Conclusion

In the tapestry of fatherhood, nurturing bonds with our children emerges as a sacred calling—a journey of love, communication, and understanding. Through the intentional investment of quality time, the cultivation of open communication, the unwavering expression of unconditional love, the exuberant cheerleading of their endeavors, and the empathetic leadership in moments of joy and strife, we forge bonds that transcend the constraints of time and circumstance.

So, let us cherish these moments, imbuing each interaction with the depth of our love and the sincerity of our understanding. For in the tender embrace of connection, we discover the true essence of fatherhood—a legacy of love that endures, nurtured by the boundless depths of our hearts.

Leading by Example: Shaping Your Children's Future

In the intricate tapestry of fatherhood, your role transcends mere authority it's a beacon of guidance that illuminates the path to your children's growth and development. In this chapter, we embark on a journey to uncover the profound impact of leading by example, exploring how your actions, attitudes, and values sculpt the very essence of your children's character and beliefs.

Modeling Integrity and Honesty

At the core of strong character lies integrity—a steadfast commitment to truthfulness and ethical conduct. As a father, your daily choices serve as a blueprint for your children's moral compass. Uphold integrity in all facets of life, demonstrating honesty and transparency even in the face of adversity. By modeling integrity, you instill in your children a deep-seated trust and integrity, cultivating a generation of individuals who uphold moral principles with unwavering resolve.

Demonstrating Respect and Kindness

Respect and kindness are the cornerstones of harmonious relationships and compassionate communities. Lead by example, showing respect for diversity and empathy for others' experiences. Model kindness in your interactions, demonstrating the transformative power of compassion and understanding. Through your actions, teach your children the invaluable lesson that every act of kindness, no matter how small, holds the potential to brighten someone's day and uplift humanity as a whole.

Teaching Responsibility and Accountability

Responsibility and accountability are the building blocks of self-reliance and personal growth. Set a positive example by fulfilling your obligations with diligence and dedication. Hold yourself accountable for your choices and actions, demonstrating resilience in the face of challenges. Through your steadfast commitment to responsibility, empower your children to embrace accountability as a guiding principle in navigating life's complexities with grace and fortitude.

Cultivating a Growth Mindset

A growth mindset fuels the flames of resilience and fosters a spirit of continuous learning and improvement. Nurture this mindset in your children by celebrating their efforts and perseverance, rather than focusing solely on outcomes. Encourage them to embrace challenges as opportunities for growth, fostering a mindset rooted in resilience and determination. By modeling a positive attitude towards setbacks and failures, you imbue your children with the transformative power of perseverance, equipping them to navigate life's twists and turns with unwavering confidence and optimism.

In essence, by leading by example, you illuminate the path to your children's future—a journey defined by integrity, respect, responsibility, and a relentless pursuit of growth. So, let your actions serve as a guiding light, inspiring and empowering your children to embrace the boundless possibilities that lie ahead with courage, compassion, and unwavering determination.

Prioritizing Self-Improvement

In the symphony of fatherhood, the melody of self-improvement resonates as a guiding principle—a testament to the relentless pursuit of growth and evolution. In this section, we delve into the transformative power of prioritizing self-improvement and its profound impact on shaping the character and aspirations of our children.

Commitment to Growth

As fathers, we are the architects of our own destiny, crafting a legacy of resilience and ambition that echoes through the corridors of time. Embrace the journey of self-improvement with fervor and determination, committing yourself to continual growth and development. Whether through further education, the pursuit of passions, or the setting and attainment of personal goals, let your children witness firsthand the transformative power of a commitment to self-improvement.

Modeling Lifelong Learning

Learning is not confined to the walls of a classroom; it's a journey that unfolds with each passing moment—an exploration of the boundless depths of knowledge and experience. Lead by example, demonstrating a voracious appetite for learning and an insatiable curiosity for the world around you. Show your children that education is a lifelong pursuit, one that enriches the mind and nourishes the soul, fostering a spirit of intellectual curiosity and discovery that will guide them throughout their lives.

Embracing Personal Growth

Personal growth is a journey of self-discovery—a voyage into the depths of one's potential and aspirations. Embrace this journey with open arms, challenging yourself to transcend limitations and surpass expectations. Set ambitious goals and pursue them with unwavering determination, demonstrating to your children the transformative power of resilience and perseverance in the pursuit of greatness.

Conclusion

In the grand tapestry of fatherhood, leading by example emerges as a beacon of guidance—a testament to the enduring legacy of integrity, kindness, responsibility, and growth. Through your actions, you sculpt a vision of possibility and purpose, inspiring and empowering your children to embark on their own journeys of self-discovery with courage and conviction.

So, let us lead by example, embracing the relentless pursuit of self-improvement with unwavering resolve and boundless enthusiasm. For in the glow of our aspirations, we ignite the flames of inspiration in the hearts of our children, illuminating the path to a future defined by limitless potential and boundless opportunity.

CHAPTER 4: Embracing Challenges

Navigating the Challenges of Fatherhood

In the tapestry of fatherhood, challenges emerge as the threads that weave resilience and fortitude into the fabric of our journey. Embracing these trials with unwavering resolve is not only essential for personal growth but also serves as a profound example for our children. In this chapter, we embark on a journey to explore the art of overcoming obstacles, navigating the delicate balance between work and family life, and fostering a spirit of resilience that illuminates the path to a brighter future.

Embracing Challenges with Resilience

Fatherhood is a journey rife with twists and turns, presenting a myriad of challenges that test the limits of our resolve. Embrace these challenges as opportunities for growth and self-discovery, knowing that with each obstacle overcome, you emerge stronger and more resilient. Teach your children the value of perseverance and determination, instilling in them a steadfast belief in their ability to overcome adversity with grace and courage.

Balancing Work and Family Life

Finding equilibrium between the demands of work and the joys of family life is a delicate dance one that requires careful planning and prioritization. Strive to strike a harmonious balance, carving out dedicated time for both professional pursuits and cherished moments with your loved ones. By modeling the importance of work-life balance, you impart invaluable lessons in time management and prioritization, nurturing a sense of harmony and fulfillment in your children's lives.

Navigating Difficult Conversations

Difficult conversations are an inevitable part of parenthood, challenging us to navigate sensitive topics with empathy and understanding. Approach these conversations with an open heart and a willingness to listen, creating a safe space for your children to express their thoughts and feelings. Show empathy and compassion, validating their emotions and offering guidance and support as they navigate life's complexities. By fostering open communication and emotional intelligence, you equip your children with the tools they need to navigate difficult conversations with confidence and grace.

Conclusion

In the grand tapestry of fatherhood, challenges emerge as the crucible in which resilience and fortitude are forged. Embrace these trials with unwavering resolve, knowing that each obstacle overcome serves as a testament to your strength and determination. By navigating the delicate balance between work and family life, fostering open communication, and modeling resilience in the face of adversity, you illuminate the path to a future defined by courage, compassion, and unwavering resilience.

Providing Support and Encouragement

In the intricate tapestry of fatherhood, the role of support and encouragement emerges as a guiding light—a beacon of strength and reassurance in the face of adversity. In this section, we delve into the transformative power of providing unwavering support and encouragement to our children, nurturing resilience and fortitude in their journey through life's challenges.

Being a Pillar of Support

Amidst life's tumultuous waves, be the steadfast anchor that grounds your children in times of uncertainty and doubt. Offer a listening ear and a shoulder to lean on, providing guidance, empathy, and reassurance during difficult times. Encourage your children to express their emotions openly, validating their feelings without judgment and offering unwavering support as they navigate the complexities of life. By being a pillar of support, you empower your children to face challenges with confidence and determination, knowing that they are not alone in their struggles.

Fostering a Culture of Encouragement

Encouragement is the nourishment that fuels the flames of resilience and determination, igniting a spark of motivation in the hearts of our children. Celebrate their efforts and progress, no matter how small, and shower them with words of praise and encouragement. Acknowledge their achievements, whether it's mastering a new skill, overcoming a challenge, or simply persevering in the face of adversity. By fostering a culture of encouragement, you instill in your children a sense of self-belief and motivation, empowering them to reach for the stars and pursue their dreams with unwavering determination.

Celebrating Successes, Big and Small

In the grand tapestry of parenthood, celebrations emerge as the vibrant threads that weave joy and fulfillment into the fabric of our journey. Celebrate your children's successes, big and small, with boundless enthusiasm and pride. Recognize the hard work and dedication that went into their achievements, and shower them with words of affirmation and praise. By celebrating successes, you reinforce your children's confidence and self-esteem, fueling their motivation to continue striving for excellence in all areas of life.

Conclusion

In essence, the art of providing support and encouragement serves as a cornerstone of effective parenting—a testament to the enduring bond of love and commitment that unites father and child. By offering unwavering support, fostering a culture of encouragement, and celebrating successes, you empower your children to navigate life's challenges with confidence, determination, and resilience. So, let us embrace our role as pillars of strength and beacons of encouragement, guiding our children through life's twists and turns with unwavering resolve and boundless optimism.

Cultivating Creativity in Your Children

In the tapestry of fatherhood, creativity emerges as the vibrant thread that weaves imagination, innovation, and self-expression into the fabric of our children's lives. In this chapter, we embark on a journey to explore the transformative power of nurturing creativity, uncovering the myriad ways in which you can inspire and support your children's imaginative endeavors.

Encouraging Exploration and Curiosity

Nurture the seeds of curiosity that lie within your children, encouraging them to embark on journeys of exploration and discovery. Provide opportunities for diverse activities, from painting and music to storytelling and building. Celebrate their unique interests and talents, fostering a spirit of inquiry and wonder that ignites their passion for learning and creativity.

Creating a Nurturing Environment

Craft a nurturing environment that serves as a fertile ground for creativity to flourish. Designate spaces within your home dedicated to artistic pursuits, stocked with a plethora of materials and resources that inspire creativity. Cultivate an atmosphere of freedom and encouragement, where your children feel empowered to express themselves creatively without inhibition or fear of judgment.

Embracing Imagination and Play

Embrace the boundless realm of imagination, where the ordinary transforms into the extraordinary and the mundane gives way to the magical. Encourage imaginative play through open-ended toys and materials that invite exploration and invention. Engage in playful adventures with your children, diving headfirst into the realms of make-believe and storytelling. Embrace the joy of creation, celebrating the limitless possibilities of the imagination.

Supporting Creative Risk-Taking

Foster a culture of creative risk-taking, where innovation thrives and failure is seen as a stepping stone to success. Encourage your children to take bold creative leaps, to explore uncharted territories, and to dare to dream beyond the confines of convention. Provide guidance and support as they navigate the creative process, offering constructive feedback and encouragement along the way. By nurturing their willingness to take risks, you empower your children to develop resilience, confidence, and a fearless spirit of innovation.

In essence, by cultivating creativity in your children, you ignite the spark of imagination that fuels their dreams and aspirations. So, let us embrace the transformative power of creativity, inspiring and supporting our children as they embark on their own journeys of self-discovery, innovation, and artistic expression.

Fostering Collaboration and Connection

In the tapestry of creativity, collaboration and connection form the vibrant threads that weave together ideas, perspectives, and visions. When children engage in collaborative endeavors, they not only pool their individual talents but also cultivate a fertile ground for innovation and mutual growth.

Encouraging collaborative efforts can take many forms. Group projects, where children work together to tackle challenges and bring ideas to life, instill a sense of shared responsibility and accomplishment. Creative workshops provide structured yet open-ended environments where children can explore diverse interests alongside their peers, sparking inspiration through collective exploration.

Moreover, collaborative storytelling ventures transport children into realms of shared imagination, where each participant contributes their unique voice to craft narratives that transcend individual imagination. These experiences foster empathy, communication skills, and the ability to build upon others' ideas an invaluable skill set that extends far beyond creative pursuits.

Yet, beyond the mere act of working together lies the essence of connection, a bond that transcends mere cooperation. Cultivating a sense of community around creativity nurtures an environment where every idea is cherished, and every voice is heard. Celebrating creativity as a collective endeavor fosters a spirit of inclusivity, where diversity of thought and expression is not only welcomed but celebrated.

By nurturing collaboration and connection, parents impart more than just creative skills to their children. They cultivate a mindset rooted in teamwork, communication, and cooperation, essential attributes for navigating the complexities of the modern world. Through collaborative ventures, children learn the art of compromise, the power of collective brainstorming, and the joy of witnessing their ideas flourish in the hands of others.

Conclusion

In the journey of raising creative children, fostering collaboration and connection stands as a cornerstone, a testament to the transformative power of shared endeavors. By nurturing an environment where ideas flow freely and connections thrive, parents ignite the spark of innovation within their children, empowering them to embrace creativity with passion and purpose.

As these young minds embark on their creative odyssey, guided by the nurturing hands of collaboration and connection, they embody the essence of creativity in its purest form, a force that transcends boundaries, empowers communities, and shapes the world anew. So, let us champion collaboration, celebrate connection, and witness the magic that unfolds when creativity flourishes in the fertile soil of shared endeavors.

Navigating Parenthood with Purpose

In this chapter, we delve into the profound significance of parenting with purpose. From establishing guiding principles for your family to prioritizing what truly matters, we'll explore how you can cultivate a clear vision for your role as a father and make meaningful contributions to your children's lives. Parenthood is a journey marked by blessings, trials, and countless opportunities for growth. Steering this journey with purpose and intentionality is crucial for creating a nurturing and enriching environment where your children can thrive. Let's embark on this exploration of the significance of navigating parenthood with purpose and uncover strategies for shaping your role as a father.

Defining Your Values and Priorities

Begin by articulating your values and priorities as a parent. Reflect on the core principles that guide your life and consider how they translate into your role as a father. Whether it's fostering love and connection, prioritizing education and personal development, or instilling values such as kindness and empathy, clarifying your values provides a compass for making decisions and setting goals that align with your vision for your family.

Setting Goals for Your Family

Next, set meaningful goals for your family that reflect your values and priorities. Whether it's dedicating more quality time together, nurturing a passion for learning, or creating a supportive environment for your children to pursue their dreams, establish clear objectives that shape your actions and decisions as a parent. Break down these goals into actionable steps and celebrate the progress your family makes along the way.

Establishing Routines and Rituals

Routines and rituals offer structure and stability amidst the whirlwind of parenting. Establish daily routines that promote health, well-being, and family bonding, such as shared meals, bedtime rituals, and outings together. Create meaningful rituals that mark special occasions, milestones, and family traditions, fostering a sense of belonging and connection within your family unit.

Practicing Mindful Parenthood

Mindful parenthood involves being present, attentive, and nonjudgmental in your interactions with your children. Cultivate mindfulness in your parenting by grounding yourself in the present moment, listening with empathy and understanding, and responding to your children with intentionality and patience. Embrace the blessings and challenges of parenting with openness and acceptance, savoring the precious moments you share with your children along the way.

By navigating parenthood with purpose, you not only enrich the lives of your children but also nurture a deeper sense of fulfillment and meaning in your role as a father. Embrace this journey with an open heart and a clear vision, knowing that your efforts today will shape the future of your family tomorrow.

Fostering Independence and Autonomy

Empowering your children to become confident, independent individuals is a cornerstone of effective parenting. By fostering their autonomy and self-reliance, you lay the groundwork for their future success and fulfillment. Encourage them to make choices, take on responsibilities, and learn from their actions. Provide opportunities for them to problem-solve, explore their interests, and follow their passions, guiding them with love and support as they navigate their own paths toward self-discovery and growth.

Cultivating Gratitude and Resilience

Gratitude and resilience are indispensable qualities that equip children to navigate life's ups and downs with grace and courage. Cultivate gratitude by encouraging your children to reflect on the blessings in their lives and express appreciation for the people and experiences that bring them joy. Teach them to count their blessings, even in challenging times, fostering a mindset of abundance and appreciation.

Likewise, foster resilience by helping your children bounce back from setbacks, view adversity as an opportunity for growth, and cultivate a positive outlook on life. Teach them to embrace challenges as learning experiences, building resilience muscles that will serve them well throughout their lives. By nurturing gratitude and resilience, you empower your children to face life's challenges with confidence and optimism.

Conclusion

Navigating parenting with purpose is a journey of intentionality, authenticity, and love. By defining your values and priorities, setting goals for your family, establishing routines and rituals, practicing mindful parenthood, fostering independence and autonomy, and cultivating gratitude and resilience, you create a nurturing and supportive environment where your children can thrive and flourish.

So, embrace the adventure of parenting with purpose and passion, knowing that each decision you make and each action you take shapes the future of your family. By nurturing your children with love, guidance, and unwavering support, you lay the foundation for a lifetime of happiness, success, and fulfillment.

Cultivating Adaptability: A Father's Guide

Adaptability stands as a precious skill, essential for both fathers and their children. From teaching them how to rebound from setbacks to instilling a growth mindset, we'll explore strategies for fostering adaptability, equipping your children to confront life's hurdles with resilience and determination. Adaptability is the ability to bounce back from adversity, to adjust to change, and to emerge stronger in the face of challenges. As a father, nurturing your children's adaptability is among the greatest gifts you can offer. In this chapter, we'll delve into the importance of instilling adaptability in your children and unveil techniques for nurturing this crucial quality.

Encouraging a Growth Mindset

A growth mindset embodies the belief that abilities and intelligence can be cultivated through effort and perseverance. Encourage your children to adopt a growth mindset by praising their efforts and resilience rather than solely focusing on their innate talents or abilities. Teach them to perceive challenges as opportunities for growth and learning, emphasizing the importance of adaptability, resilience, and the willingness to try again after setbacks.

Fostering Problem-Solving Skills

Problem-solving skills are vital for navigating life's obstacles with confidence and adaptability. Encourage your children to approach problems with creativity, flexibility, and resourcefulness. Teach them to break down complex problems into manageable steps, brainstorm potential solutions, and evaluate their effectiveness. Provide opportunities for them to apply problem-solving in real-life scenarios, guiding and supporting them as they hone this invaluable skill.

Promoting Emotional Regulation

Emotional regulation entails managing and expressing emotions in healthy and constructive ways. Assist your children in developing emotional regulation skills by teaching them to identify and label their feelings, understand the triggers that elicit emotional responses, and employ coping strategies to regulate their emotions. Demonstrate healthy emotional expression and coping mechanisms, and create a safe and supportive environment where your children feel comfortable expressing their emotions openly and seeking support when needed.

Cultivating Optimism and Positive Outlook

Optimism entails the belief that positive outcomes are attainable even in the face of adversity. Cultivate optimism in your children by focusing on the positives in every situation, highlighting their strengths and capabilities, and encouraging them to maintain a positive outlook on life. Teach them to reframe negative experiences and setbacks as opportunities for growth and learning, and model optimism in your own attitudes and actions.

By nurturing adaptability in your children through these strategies, you equip them with the resilience and mindset needed to navigate life's challenges with courage and determination. As a father, your guidance and support pave the way for your children to flourish and thrive, embodying the spirit of adaptability in every aspect of their lives.

Encouraging Social Support and Connection

Social support and connection serve as crucial pillars in navigating life's challenges. Encourage your children to cultivate strong connections with family members, friends, teachers, and other supportive adults. Teach them the importance of seeking help and support when needed, and demonstrate healthy communication and conflict resolution skills in your own relationships. Foster a sense of belonging and community within your family, emphasizing the value of empathy, kindness, and cooperation in building resilient and supportive connections with others.

Conclusion

Fostering adaptability in your children is a journey of commitment, growth, and self-discovery. By encouraging a growth mindset, fostering problem-solving skills, promoting emotional regulation, cultivating optimism and positive thinking, and encouraging social support and connection, you equip your children with the tools they need to navigate life's challenges with courage, adaptability, and confidence. So, nurture their adaptability with love and support, and witness as they thrive in the face of adversity, emerging stronger and more resilient than ever before.

Celebrating Milestones: A Father's Guide

Life's journey is punctuated by milestones—significant moments that mark our growth, achievements, and successes. As a father, celebrating these milestones with your children is vital to acknowledging their progress, instilling confidence, and creating lasting memories. In this chapter, we'll delve into the importance of celebrating milestones and explore meaningful ways to recognize these special occasions.

Feting Achievements, Big and Small

Every achievement, whether monumental or minuscule, deserves recognition and celebration. Whether it's mastering a new skill, reaching a personal goal, or overcoming a challenge, take the time to applaud and celebrate your children's accomplishments. Offer words of praise and encouragement, expressing pride in their dedication and perseverance. By celebrating their achievements, you bolster their confidence and motivation to continue striving for excellence.

Marking Milestones with Rituals and Traditions

Rituals and traditions play a significant role in commemorating milestones and fostering a sense of continuity and connection within families. Establish meaningful rituals to mark important milestones, such as birthdays, graduations, and milestones in personal growth and development. Whether it's a special family dinner, a heartfelt toast, or a cherished tradition passed down through generations, rituals provide a sense of stability and belonging and create lasting memories that your children will treasure for years to come.

Creating Memory Books and Keepsakes

Capture the magic of milestones by creating memory books and keepsakes that document your children's growth and achievements over the years. Take photographs, write letters, and collect mementos that encapsulate the essence of each milestone, from their first steps to their high school graduation. Create scrapbooks, memory boxes, or digital albums to preserve these precious memories, revisiting them together as a family to reminisce and celebrate how far they've come.

Planning Special Outings and Events

Celebrate milestones with special outings and events that create lasting memories and strengthen family bonds. Plan a day trip to a favorite destination, organize a family adventure, or treat your children to a special outing or experience they've been dreaming of. Whether it's a day at the beach, a visit to a museum, or a thrilling adventure park, the time spent together creating new memories will be cherished for years to come.

By celebrating milestones in these meaningful ways, you not only acknowledge your children's achievements but also create enduring bonds and cherished memories that will last a lifetime. As a father, your role in commemorating these milestones is invaluable, shaping the narrative of your family's journey and creating a legacy of love, support, and celebration.

Incorporating Reflection and Gratitude

Milestones serve as opportunities for reflection and gratitude, not only for the progress your children have made but also for the love and support that surround them. Encourage your children to reflect on their achievements, express gratitude for the individuals who have supported them along the journey, and set intentions for the future. Create space for meaningful conversations and genuine expressions of appreciation, celebrating the journey of growth and discovery together as a family.

Conclusion

Celebrating milestones is a joyful and meaningful way to acknowledge the progress, achievements, and successes of your children. By commemorating their accomplishments, marking milestones with rituals and traditions, creating memory books and keepsakes, planning special outings and events, and incorporating reflection and gratitude, you foster a culture of celebration and support that nurtures their confidence, adaptability, and sense of belonging. So, celebrate each milestone with love and enthusiasm, and witness as your children continue to thrive and flourish on their journey through life.

Fatherhood: A Journey of Growth and Evolution

Fatherhood is a dynamic voyage, an ongoing exploration of growth and transformation. In this concluding chapter, we'll reflect on the lessons learned and the joys experienced along the way. From embracing change to adapting to the needs of your growing family, we'll explore how you can continue to excel as a dad, regardless of what the future may hold.

Embracing Evolution in Fatherhood

Fatherhood today is a multifaceted journey, shaped by shifting societal norms and individual experiences. Embracing this evolution is crucial for fathers to adapt, grow, and thrive in their roles as caregivers, mentors, and role models. Explore the significance of embracing fatherhood's evolution, navigating the changing dynamics of parenthood with grace and resilience.

Adapting to Changing Roles and Responsibilities

Modern fatherhood encompasses a diverse array of roles and responsibilities beyond traditional gender norms. Embrace this evolution by adapting to changing roles within your family dynamic. Whether it's sharing caregiving duties, participating actively in household tasks, or supporting your partner's career aspirations, be open to redefining what it means to be a father in today's world.

Navigating Technology and Digital Parenting

Technology has revolutionized the parenting landscape, presenting both opportunities and challenges for fathers. Embrace technology as a tool for connection, learning, and creativity while setting boundaries and modeling healthy screen habits for your children. Stay informed about online safety and digital literacy, engaging in open conversations with your children about responsible technology use.

Cultivating Emotional Intelligence and Vulnerability

Foster emotional intelligence and vulnerability as essential qualities of modern fatherhood. Cultivate open communication and create a safe space for your children to express their emotions freely. Model vulnerability by sharing your own feelings and experiences, encouraging empathy, compassion, and resilience in navigating emotions and relationships.

Supporting Work-Life Integration

Balancing professional responsibilities with family life is a common challenge for fathers. Embrace the task of work-life integration by prioritizing quality time with your family, setting boundaries between work and home life, and seeking support from your employer and community resources. Foster a culture of flexibility and understanding that allows you to fulfill your commitments both at work and at home.

As you continue on your journey of fatherhood, remember that growth and evolution are inherent parts of the process. Embrace change, adapt to new roles and responsibilities, and cultivate meaningful connections with your children and family. With resilience, compassion, and dedication, you'll continue to rock as a dad, creating cherished memories and shaping the future for generations to come.

Championing Diversity, Equity, and Inclusion

As fatherhood continues to evolve, there's a growing recognition of the importance of diversity, equity, and inclusion in parenting practices and family structures. Embrace diversity in all its facets, celebrating the unique identities and experiences of your children, and fostering an environment of inclusivity and acceptance within your family and community. Advocate for equitable policies and resources that support all families, irrespective of race, ethnicity, gender, or socioeconomic status.

Celebrating Diversity and Inclusivity

Recognize and celebrate the diversity within your family and community. Embrace different cultures, traditions, and perspectives, and teach your children to respect and appreciate the richness of diversity. Encourage them to be curious, open-minded, and empathetic towards others, fostering a sense of belonging and inclusivity for all.

Promoting Equity and Access

Advocate for equitable opportunities and resources for all children, regardless of their background or circumstances. Support initiatives that promote equal access to education, healthcare, and other essential services, and challenge systemic barriers that perpetuate inequality and discrimination. Lead by example by treating everyone with fairness, respect, and dignity, and instill in your children the values of justice, compassion, and empathy.

Creating Inclusive Spaces

Create inclusive spaces within your family and community where everyone feels valued, respected, and heard. Encourage open dialogue and meaningful conversations about diversity, equity, and inclusion, and challenge stereotypes and biases that perpetuate discrimination. Take proactive steps to address inequality and promote social justice, both within your immediate surroundings and in the broader society.

Conclusion

Embracing fatherhood's evolution is a journey of self-discovery, growth, and transformation. By adapting to changing roles and responsibilities, navigating technology and digital parenting, cultivating emotional intelligence and vulnerability, supporting work-life integration, and championing diversity, equity, and inclusion, you empower yourself to thrive as a modern father and create a nurturing and supportive environment for your children to flourish. So, embrace the journey of fatherhood with an open heart and an open mind, and watch as your family grows stronger and closer with each new chapter.

SUMMARY

Rock Solid: A Guide to Being the Dad Your Kids Need stands as a practical and insightful roadmap for fathers striving to cultivate strong relationships with their children. Authored by Robert A. Reader, this book delves into the essential qualities and actions that define a father as a positive and influential figure in the lives of his kids.

Reader underscores the paramount importance of being present and actively engaged in every phase of a child's life, from infancy through adulthood. He stresses the significance of embodying a consistent role model, providing unwavering support, guidance, and unconditional love. Through a blend of personal anecdotes and actionable advice, Reader illustrates how fathers can forge trust, communicate effectively, and impart values that will shape their children's character.

The book traverses a spectrum of topics including discipline, setting boundaries, nurturing emotional intelligence, and surmounting challenges unique to fatherhood. It urges fathers to embrace their role with confidence and intentionality, acknowledging the profound impact they wield on their children's development and well-being.

Rock Solid serves as an invaluable compass for fathers eager to fortify their connections with their children and establish an enduring legacy of love, guidance, and support. It furnishes practical strategies and timeless wisdom to assist fathers in navigating the joys and trials of parenthood, ultimately empowering them to embody the fathers their children require and deserve.

CONCLUSION

Rock Solid: A Guide to Being the Dad Your Kids Need transcends mere pages,it serves as a comprehensive roadmap for fathers dedicated to leaving a lasting, positive imprint on their children's lives. More than a simple read, it's an invitation to action, a call to arms for fathers everywhere to step up and make a meaningful impact in the lives of their children.

So, seize a copy of this invaluable guide, prepare to dive in headfirst, and get ready to roll up your sleeves and embark on the journey of fatherhood with newfound purpose and determination. With Rock Solid as your guide, you'll be equipped with the tools, insights, and inspiration needed to rock as a dad and nurture strong, enduring bonds with your children.